SUZANNE BYRD

Wired for Love

Embracing ADHD and Building Intimate Connections

Copyright © 2024 by Suzanne Byrd

All rights reserved. No part of this publication may be reproduced, stored or transmitted in any form or by any means, electronic, mechanical, photocopying, recording, scanning, or otherwise without written permission from the publisher. It is illegal to copy this book, post it to a website, or distribute it by any other means without permission.

First edition

This book was professionally typeset on Reedsy. Find out more at reedsy.com

Contents

1. Understanding ADHD Through a Woman's Lens   1
2. The ADHD Mind and the Foundations of Intimacy   9
3. Love Languages, ADHD, and Emotional Connection   18
4. ADHD, Intimacy, and Sensory Overload   26
5. Communication Struggles and Strengths in ADHD Relationships   35
6. Navigating the Roller Coaster of Emotional Intensity   43
7. The Hormonal Puzzle   52
8. Parenthood, ADHD, and Relationship Dynamics   59
9. Leveraging ADHD Strengths for Deeper Connections   68
10. Healing, Growth, and Thriving Together   76

1

Understanding ADHD Through a Woman's Lens

For many women, the journey of discovering they have ADHD feels like uncovering a missing puzzle piece. Society has long associated ADHD with hyperactive boys, leaving countless women to navigate a world that misjudges their challenges as character flaws or failures. Yet, ADHD in women is not just a lesser-known narrative—it is a profoundly different experience. Understanding how it manifests in women is the first step toward creating deeper connections and fulfilling relationships.

—-

The ADHD Spectrum: How Women Are Different

ADHD in women often goes undiagnosed or misdiagnosed for years. Unlike the stereotypical hyperactive child, women with ADHD are more likely to internalize their struggles. They might seem daydreamy, overly emotional, or perpetually overwhelmed. These differences can be traced back to how ADHD symptoms manifest in more subtle or socially acceptable ways in girls and women.

Women with ADHD often face challenges like:

Emotional Dysregulation: Heightened emotions that can swing rapidly from joy to frustration.

Perfectionism and Shame: A constant feeling of not being "good enough" despite immense effort.

Masking and Overcompensating: A tendency to hide symptoms and work excessively to appear competent.

Executive Function Challenges: Struggles with organization, time management, and maintaining routines.

In relationships, these traits can lead to misunderstandings. A partner might see their loved one's distraction as disinterest or their emotional intensity as unpredictability, when in fact these are manifestations of ADHD.

—-

Emotional Intensity and ADHD Relationships

One hallmark of ADHD in women is emotional intensity. This intensity can manifest as:

1. Rejection Sensitivity Dysphoria (RSD): A deep fear of rejection or criticism, often leading to overthinking or avoidance behaviors.

2. Hyperfocus on Relationships: Women with ADHD may become deeply invested in their partners, often prioritizing their needs over their own.

3. Emotional Overflow: A tendency to feel emotions so deeply that they can't be easily processed or articulated.

While these traits can create challenges, they also come with strengths. Women with ADHD are often passionate, empathetic, and fiercely loyal. They bring unique energy and creativity to their relationships, which can lead to powerful bonds when understood and nurtured.

—-

Case Study: Mia's Journey to Understanding

Mia, a 34-year-old graphic designer, had always struggled in relationships. She found herself overwhelmed by minor disagreements, often feeling rejected even when her partner reassured her otherwise. In one relationship, her boyfriend accused her of being "needy" and overly emotional. Mia couldn't explain why she felt the way she did, but she knew her reactions were disproportionate to the situation.

When Mia was diagnosed with ADHD, she finally understood the patterns that had dominated her life. Her emotional intensity wasn't a flaw—it was a part of her brain's wiring. With therapy and self-awareness, she began learning tools to manage her emotions and communicate her needs more effectively. In her next relationship, Mia openly discussed her ADHD with her partner, allowing them to navigate challenges together.

This journey of understanding transformed Mia's relationships—not just with others, but with herself.

—-

Key Challenges Women with ADHD Face in Relationships

1. Inconsistency: Partners may struggle with the ADHD individual's tendency to hyperfocus on one aspect of the relationship while neglecting others.

2. Forgetfulness: Important dates, tasks, or conversations may slip through the cracks, leading to frustration.

3. Emotional Volatility: Heightened sensitivity can lead to frequent conflicts or miscommunication.

4. Impulsivity: Making decisions or reacting without thinking can strain trust and stability.

Understanding these challenges isn't about blame—it's about creating strategies to overcome them. Many women with ADHD find that their relationships improve dramatically when both partners recognize these traits and work together to address them.

—-

The Overlap of ADHD and Gender Expectations

Gender roles play a significant part in how ADHD impacts women. Society often expects women to be the emotional caregivers, the organizers, and the peacemakers in relationships. These expectations can be overwhelming for someone with ADHD, who may already struggle with executive function and emotional regulation.

For example:

A woman with ADHD might feel immense guilt for forgetting her partner's birthday or for struggling to keep the house tidy.

She may overextend herself in an attempt to "prove" her worth, leading to burnout and resentment.

In heterosexual relationships, her partner might unknowingly reinforce these dynamics by expecting her to shoulder the majority of emotional labor.

Recognizing and dismantling these expectations is crucial for creating healthier, more equitable relationships.

—-

Strengths ADHD Women Bring to Relationships

Despite the challenges, women with ADHD bring incredible strengths to their relationships. These include:

1. Creativity: They often think outside the box, bringing fresh ideas and energy to problem-solving.

2. Passion: Their emotional intensity can translate into deep love and dedication.

3. Empathy: Many ADHD women are highly attuned to their partner's feelings and needs.

4. Spontaneity: Their adventurous spirit can keep relationships exciting and dynamic.

Learning to harness these strengths can help women with ADHD build fulfilling, resilient partnerships.

—-

Practical Takeaways for Women and Their Partners

Self-Awareness is Key: Understanding your ADHD traits is the first step toward navigating relationships effectively. Journaling, therapy, and self-reflection can help.

Open Communication: Be honest with your partner about your ADHD and how it affects your relationship. Discuss your needs and challenges openly.

Celebrate Small Wins: Focus on the positive aspects of your relationship and acknowledge the progress you've made together.

For partners, empathy and patience are crucial. Instead of viewing ADHD traits as faults, recognize them as part of what makes your loved one unique. Together, you can create a relationship that embraces both strengths and challenges.

—-

Embracing the ADHD Lens

ADHD is not a deficit—it's a different way of experiencing the world. For women, understanding how this lens shapes their emotions, behaviors, and relationships is the foundation for growth and connection. By embracing their unique traits and working collaboratively with their partners, women with ADHD can build intimate relationships that are both meaningful and rewarding.

This journey begins with self-compassion and a willingness to explore what works for you—and Chapter 2 will delve deeper into how ADHD minds build the foundations of intimacy.

2

The ADHD Mind and the Foundations of Intimacy

Building Relationships with an ADHD Brain

Intimacy is not just about physical closeness; it's about connection, trust, and understanding. For women with ADHD, these foundational elements of relationships can feel elusive. Challenges like emotional dysregulation, impulsivity, or forgetfulness may create friction. Yet, beneath these hurdles lies a unique potential for deep, meaningful bonds.

To build intimacy, women with ADHD must navigate their relationships with intention, honesty, and creativity—starting with understanding how their minds shape connection.

—-

Attachment Styles and ADHD

Attachment theory offers a lens for understanding how we approach intimacy. Our attachment style—whether secure, anxious, avoidant, or disorganized—forms in childhood and continues to influence our relationships. For women with ADHD, these dynamics can become more pronounced:

Anxious Attachment: Often fueled by rejection sensitivity dysphoria (RSD), women with ADHD may crave constant reassurance, fearing abandonment even in stable relationships.

Avoidant Attachment: Overwhelmed by emotional demands, some women might retreat into solitude, struggling to engage fully in their relationships.

Disorganized Attachment: A mix of seeking closeness and pushing it away, driven by confusion and emotional volatility.

The good news is that attachment styles aren't fixed. By understanding their own tendencies, women with ADHD can work toward building secure, supportive connections.

—-

Case Study: Sarah's Struggle with Reassurance

Sarah, a 29-year-old teacher, often found herself seeking constant reassurance from her partner, James. If he didn't text back immediately, she assumed he was upset or losing interest. Her anxiety would spiral into emotional outbursts, leaving James confused and overwhelmed.

After learning about RSD and her anxious attachment style, Sarah started recognizing her triggers. She began journaling her fears instead of immediately confronting James, giving herself time to process her emotions. She also shared her struggles with James, who responded with patience and understanding. Together, they established ways to communicate that reassured Sarah without placing undue pressure on James.

Trust and Vulnerability: Overcoming ADHD Challenges

Building trust and being vulnerable are cornerstones of intimacy, but ADHD traits can sometimes get in the way.

1. Inconsistency and Follow-Through: Forgetfulness or being easily distracted can make a partner feel de-prioritized.

2. Emotional Overreaction: Misinterpreting neutral actions as criticism or rejection can lead to conflict.

3. Impulsivity: Saying or doing things in the heat of the moment can strain trust.

The key to overcoming these challenges lies in self-awareness and clear communication:

Own Your Challenges: Acknowledge when ADHD behaviors—like forgetting an anniversary or zoning out during a conversation—affect your partner. Apologizing and explaining can go a long way in rebuilding trust.

Create Systems for Consistency: Use reminders, shared calendars, or rituals to ensure reliability in your relationship.

Pause Before Reacting: When emotions run high, take a moment to reflect before responding.

— -

Emotional Regulation and Connection

Women with ADHD often feel emotions more intensely than others. This intensity can be both a gift and a challenge. While it allows for profound empathy and passion, it can also overwhelm partners who may not share the same emotional bandwidth.

To regulate emotions and foster connection:

Practice Mindfulness: Techniques like deep breathing or grounding exercises can help manage overwhelming feelings.

Use "I" Statements: Express emotions without blaming your

partner (e.g., "I feel anxious when plans change suddenly" instead of "You never stick to plans").

Seek Outside Support: Therapy, coaching, or ADHD support groups can offer tools and validation.

Case Study: Maria and the Emotional Roller Coaster

Maria, a 38-year-old artist, described her emotions as a "tidal wave." Small disagreements with her wife, Nina, often spiraled into intense arguments. Maria felt deeply misunderstood, while Nina felt drained by the constant emotional flux.

Through therapy, Maria began identifying her triggers and practicing grounding techniques. Nina learned to approach Maria's emotional moments with curiosity instead of defensiveness. Over time, they established a pattern of "pausing" during conflicts to reset their conversation, creating a more balanced dynamic.

Building a Foundation of Trust: Practical Strategies

1. Be Transparent About ADHD: Sharing how ADHD affects your thoughts, feelings, and behaviors can foster understanding and

patience.

2. Create Rituals of Connection: Establish small, consistent habits that strengthen your bond, like a weekly date night or morning check-ins.

3. Use Visual or Physical Cues: For example, leaving a sticky note reminder to pick up a partner's favorite snack can demonstrate thoughtfulness even when your mind feels scattered.

4. Celebrate Progress: Acknowledge growth in your relationship, even in small ways, to reinforce positive patterns.

—-

Communication as a Pillar of Intimacy

Women with ADHD may struggle with communication due to:

Interrupting or Forgetting Details: Impulsivity can lead to speaking out of turn, while poor working memory can make following conversations challenging.

Misinterpreting Tone or Intent: Rejection sensitivity can cause women to read negativity into neutral comments.

Over-Talking or Hyperfocusing: Some partners may feel overshadowed when their ADHD partner dominates a conversation or fixates on a single topic.

To improve communication:

Practice Active Listening: Summarize what your partner says to ensure you understand before responding.

Set Boundaries for Conversations: Schedule discussions for times when you're calm and focused.

Address Conflicts Head-On: Avoid letting misunderstandings fester by addressing them early with kindness and clarity.

—-

The Role of Forgiveness in ADHD Relationships

Because ADHD traits can sometimes lead to unintended hurt, forgiveness is a critical part of any relationship involving ADHD. Forgiveness, however, doesn't mean overlooking issues—it means working together to grow from them.

For Yourself: Let go of guilt over past mistakes and focus on how you can improve moving forward.

For Your Partner: Recognize their efforts to understand and

support you, even when they don't get it right.

Case Study: Sophie and the Missed Anniversary

Sophie, a 41-year-old with ADHD, forgot her partner Liam's birthday despite setting multiple reminders. Liam felt hurt, interpreting the oversight as a lack of care. Sophie, meanwhile, spiraled into guilt and shame, worrying she had irreparably damaged their relationship.

To rebuild trust, Sophie apologized sincerely, explaining that her ADHD made remembering dates difficult despite her best efforts. She also made a plan to celebrate Liam's birthday that weekend, showing her commitment to making amends. Liam, understanding the role of ADHD, forgave Sophie and appreciated her effort to repair the situation.

Building Intimacy Step by Step

Creating intimacy as a woman with ADHD isn't about eliminating every challenge—it's about recognizing them and finding ways to navigate them together. By understanding their own minds and embracing tools for connection, women with ADHD can lay the groundwork for relationships that thrive on trust, understanding, and love.

Chapter 3 will explore how ADHD women can navigate love languages and emotional connection, offering creative ways to strengthen their bonds with partners.

3

Love Languages, ADHD, and Emotional Connection

The Language of Love

Love is expressed and received in countless ways, yet many relationships falter because partners speak different "love languages." Dr. Gary Chapman's concept of the five love languages—words of affirmation, quality time, physical touch, acts of service, and receiving gifts—has become a cornerstone of understanding connection.

For women with ADHD, love languages can be both a lifeline and a challenge. While ADHD traits might make some expressions of love more difficult, they also offer unique opportunities for creativity and authenticity in building emotional bonds. This chapter explores how women with ADHD can navigate their love languages and those of their partners to create deeper intimacy.

—-

ADHD and the Love Languages

1. Words of Affirmation

Women with ADHD often experience rejection sensitivity dysphoria (RSD), making words of affirmation particularly meaningful—or harmful. A kind word can lift their spirits, while a careless comment can linger for days.

Challenge: Forgetting to verbalize appreciation or overanalyzing a partner's words.

Opportunity: ADHD creativity can turn affirmations into heartfelt letters, playful notes, or spontaneous compliments.

2. Quality Time

Quality time means focused attention, which can be difficult for ADHD brains prone to distraction. While ADHD women may deeply value shared moments, staying present in them can be a challenge.

Challenge: Being distracted by phones, to-do lists, or wandering thoughts during time together.

Opportunity: Hyperfocus can turn a shared activity into a magical, immersive experience.

3. Physical Touch

For some women with ADHD, physical touch is grounding and comforting. For others, sensory sensitivities can make it overwhelming or inconsistent.

Challenge: Sensory overload may make physical intimacy difficult during high-stress periods.
Opportunity: Experimenting with touch, from gentle hand-holding to deeper physical connection, can open new avenues of intimacy.

4. Acts of Service
Acts of service—doing something thoughtful for a partner—can strengthen bonds, but ADHD-related forgetfulness or executive function challenges may make consistency difficult.

Challenge: Overpromising and underdelivering on commitments, leading to feelings of guilt or frustration.
Opportunity: Turning small, achievable tasks into meaningful gestures of love.

5. Receiving Gifts
ADHD brains thrive on novelty, making gifts an exciting way to express love. However, the impulsivity associated with ADHD may lead to financial strain or misaligned priorities.

Challenge: Forgetting important occasions or impulsively buying impractical gifts.

Opportunity: Creative and personalized gift-giving that reflects thoughtfulness and care.

Case Study: Emma and Jake's Love Language Misalignment

Emma, a 33-year-old with ADHD, felt loved when Jake helped her with tasks like cooking or organizing her chaotic workspace. However, Jake's love language was quality time, and he often felt neglected when Emma became distracted during their evenings together.

After learning about love languages, Emma and Jake began addressing their differences. Emma used her ADHD creativity to plan small, uninterrupted activities, like board games or walks, that allowed her to stay present with Jake. In turn, Jake started helping Emma with her morning routine, an act of service that made her feel supported and loved.

Strategies for Navigating Love Languages with ADHD

1. Identify Your Love Language(s): ADHD women often feel connected to more than one love language. Use tools like quizzes or reflective journaling to pinpoint what makes you feel most loved.

2. Share Your Needs: ADHD can make it hard to articulate needs, but open conversations about love languages help partners meet each other halfway. Be specific: "I feel loved when you compliment me on my work" is clearer than "I need more support."

3. Create Systems for Follow-Through: Use calendars, reminders, or sticky notes to stay on top of love language expressions like remembering special dates or planning quality time.

—-

Creative Approaches to Love Languages for ADHD Women

Words of Affirmation: Keep a "praise journal" where you jot down compliments or affirmations your partner gives you. On days when RSD flares up, revisit these notes for reassurance.

Quality Time: Use ADHD-friendly tools like fidget toys or engaging activities to help you stay present during shared moments.

Physical Touch: Explore what types of touch feel grounding versus overstimulating. Communicate your preferences openly with your partner.

Acts of Service: Start small. For example, surprise your partner by making their coffee or tidying a shared space.

Receiving Gifts: Use ADHD creativity to craft personalized gifts like a playlist, photo album, or handmade card.

—-

Case Study: Lily's Journey with Words of Affirmation

Lily, a 27-year-old with ADHD, often felt anxious about whether her partner, Sam, appreciated her. Sam wasn't naturally expressive, and his quiet demeanor left Lily feeling unloved.

After discussing love languages, Sam began leaving sticky notes around their apartment with simple affirmations like "You're amazing" or "Thanks for making me laugh." For Lily, these small gestures transformed their relationship. She, in turn, began giving Sam affirmations in his love language: heartfelt texts and verbal praise during conversations.

—-

Love Languages as a Pathway to Emotional Connection

Emotional connection often grows from consistent, intentional acts of love. For ADHD women, this means working with their unique traits to build meaningful rituals. These rituals don't have to be grand; they can be as simple as:

A nightly check-in to share something positive from the day.

A shared playlist for long car rides or cleaning sessions.

A weekly ritual, like Sunday morning coffee or Friday movie nights, to ensure uninterrupted quality time.

—-

Navigating Misalignment in Love Languages

Partners often speak different love languages, which can lead to misunderstandings. ADHD women may feel disheartened when their efforts aren't recognized or reciprocated. To bridge this gap:

1. Be Patient: Love languages aren't always intuitive, especially for neurotypical partners unfamiliar with ADHD.

2. Educate Your Partner: Share resources about ADHD and love languages to foster empathy and understanding.

3. Acknowledge Small Efforts: Celebrate even imperfect attempts to express love in your language.

—-

Case Study: Navigating Gifts with ADHD

Maya, a 36-year-old with ADHD, loved giving gifts but often

forgot important dates like her partner Tom's birthday. One year, she impulsively bought a gift the night before, which left Tom feeling unappreciated.

Determined to improve, Maya set up a system using her phone's calendar. She scheduled reminders two weeks before special occasions and brainstormed thoughtful gifts in advance. Tom, recognizing her effort, began appreciating Maya's quirky and creative approach to gift-giving.

—-

Love Languages as Bridges to Intimacy

For women with ADHD, love languages offer a powerful framework for navigating intimacy. By understanding their own needs and creatively meeting their partner's, they can build deeper emotional connections.

Chapter 4 will delve into the sensory world of ADHD and its impact on physical intimacy, exploring how women can create comfortable, fulfilling experiences with their partners.

4

ADHD, Intimacy, and Sensory Overload

The Sensory Experience of ADHD

For many women with ADHD, intimacy isn't just an emotional experience—it's also a sensory one. ADHD brains are wired to be hyperaware of sensory input, which can range from the soothing to the overwhelming. This heightened sensitivity plays a significant role in physical intimacy, shaping how women engage with touch, sound, smell, and their environment during intimate moments.

While sensory overload can create challenges, understanding these reactions can empower women to create intimate experiences that feel safe, enjoyable, and deeply connected.

—-

The ADHD Sensory Spectrum

ADHD impacts sensory processing, often making the world feel more intense. For physical intimacy, this can manifest as:

1. Hyper-Sensitivity: A heightened awareness of touch, sound, or smell that can feel pleasurable or overwhelming.

2. Under-Sensitivity: A reduced sensory response, leading to a need for stronger or more varied stimuli to feel engaged.

3. Sensory Overload: A state where too much input—such as light, noise, or a rough fabric—becomes unbearable, shutting down the ability to enjoy intimacy.

—-

The Intersection of Sensory Needs and Physical Intimacy

For women with ADHD, sensory challenges can influence physical closeness in profound ways:

Touch: While some find certain types of touch deeply grounding, others may feel discomfort or even irritation from sensations that are too light or persistent.

Environment: Bright lights, cluttered spaces, or loud noises can distract or overwhelm, pulling focus away from connection.

Mood and Energy Levels: Sensory preferences may fluctuate

with hormonal changes, fatigue, or emotional states, making consistency difficult.

These dynamics can confuse partners who misinterpret sensory reactions as rejection.

— -

Case Study: Aisha's Struggle with Touch

Aisha, a 32-year-old graphic designer, loved holding hands with her partner, Ellie, but struggled with more prolonged physical touch. Ellie often felt hurt, assuming Aisha was uncomfortable with intimacy.

Through reflection, Aisha realized that certain fabrics and textures overstimulated her skin, making touch feel unpleasant rather than soothing. She communicated this to Ellie, who started using soft blankets and experimenting with gentler forms of touch. By addressing Aisha's sensory needs, they transformed a point of tension into a new way to connect.

— -

Strategies for Navigating Sensory Overload in Intimacy

1. Identify Your Sensory Triggers: Reflect on the types of sensations that feel good versus those that feel overwhelming.

2. Communicate Openly: Share your sensory preferences with your partner, framing them as part of what makes intimacy enjoyable for you.

3. Create a Sensory-Friendly Environment: Make small changes to your space, like dimming lights, using soothing scents, or playing soft music.

—-

Creating a Safe Sensory Space for Intimacy

1. Lighting: Avoid harsh overhead lights. Opt for warm, adjustable lighting like lamps or candles.

2. Temperature: Ensure the room feels comfortable—too hot or cold can be distracting.

3. Texture: Choose soft, smooth fabrics for bedding or clothing. Scratchy materials can ruin the experience.

4. Sound: Use calming playlists or white noise machines to block out disruptive sounds.

These adjustments help create an environment where you feel safe, relaxed, and ready to connect.

—-

Case Study: Rachel's Sensory Sanctuary

Rachel, a 40-year-old mother of two, found intimacy challenging after long days filled with sensory input from her children and work. By the time her husband, Alex, initiated physical closeness, Rachel often felt overwhelmed and distant.

Together, they designed a sensory sanctuary in their bedroom. They decluttered the space, invested in soft linens, and added a diffuser with lavender oil. Rachel also started taking short "sensory reset" breaks after work, allowing her to decompress before connecting with Alex. These changes revitalized their physical intimacy.

—-

Grounding Touch and ADHD

Touch can be both grounding and stimulating for ADHD women. To make touch feel safe and enjoyable:

Experiment with Pressure: Some women prefer firm, grounding pressure (like a weighted blanket or massage), while others enjoy light, playful touch.

Set Boundaries: Be clear about what types of touch are okay and when. For example, "I love hugs, but I need space when I'm overstimulated."

Use Tools: Sensory-friendly tools like soft brushes, textured stress balls, or cozy blankets can enhance touch experiences.

The Role of Hormones in Sensory Sensitivity

Hormonal fluctuations can amplify sensory sensitivity, especially during:

The Menstrual Cycle: Many women experience heightened touch sensitivity or irritability during PMS.

Pregnancy or Postpartum: Hormonal shifts can change sensory preferences dramatically.

Perimenopause or Menopause: Declining estrogen levels may exacerbate sensory discomfort.

Tracking these cycles can help women anticipate and adapt to changing sensory needs.

The Balance Between Sensory Overload and Emotional Intimacy

ADHD often creates a push-pull dynamic between sensory overload and the desire for emotional connection. Women with ADHD may deeply crave closeness yet feel trapped or overstimulated in the moment. To balance these needs:

1. Start Small: Begin with non-intrusive forms of touch, like sitting close together or holding hands, to build comfort.

2. Pause When Needed: If you feel overwhelmed, take a break and return to intimacy when you're ready.

3. Explore Alternatives: Intimacy doesn't always have to mean physical touch. Eye contact, shared laughter, or verbal affirmations can be equally meaningful.

—-

Case Study: Navigating Overload in New Relationships

Sofia, a 25-year-old with ADHD, struggled with physical closeness in her new relationship with Daniel. On their third date, she felt panicked when he placed his hand on her back, despite liking him deeply. Sofia's therapist helped her understand that her sensory response wasn't about Daniel—it was about her body feeling overwhelmed.

When Sofia explained this to Daniel, he responded with compassion. They experimented with slower, gentler forms of physical connection, which helped Sofia feel safe and relaxed.

— -

Celebrating Sensory Strengths in Intimacy

While sensory challenges can complicate intimacy, they also bring unique strengths:

Heightened Pleasure: When sensory experiences align with preferences, they can feel intensely pleasurable.

Attention to Detail: ADHD women often notice subtle sensations, creating opportunities for meaningful connection.

Creativity: Sensory exploration can open doors to fun, adventurous ways of connecting.

By focusing on these strengths, women with ADHD can embrace their sensory experiences as a gift rather than a limitation.

— -

Embracing Sensory Connection

Sensory preferences are an integral part of intimacy, especially for women with ADHD. By understanding their sensory needs and communicating them openly, women can transform challenges into opportunities for connection.

Chapter 5 will dive into the communication struggles and

strengths in ADHD relationships, exploring tools to foster clarity, understanding, and emotional intimacy.

5

Communication Struggles and Strengths in ADHD Relationships

The Challenge of Being Understood

For women with ADHD, communication is often the linchpin of intimacy. Misunderstandings, impulsive reactions, or zoning out during conversations can strain even the strongest relationships. Yet, ADHD also brings unique strengths to communication—creativity, passion, and empathy. The key lies in leveraging these strengths while addressing the challenges that ADHD presents.

This chapter explores how women with ADHD can improve their communication skills and build deeper connections with their partners.

—-

Understanding ADHD's Impact on Communication

ADHD traits can shape communication in several ways:

1. Impulsivity: Interrupting or speaking without filtering thoughts can lead to miscommunication or hurt feelings.

2. Forgetfulness: Missing key details of past conversations may make partners feel ignored or unimportant.

3. Emotional Dysregulation: Reacting with intensity, even when the situation doesn't warrant it, can escalate conflicts unnecessarily.

4. Distractibility: Zoning out or losing focus during important discussions may create frustration for both parties.

While these tendencies can create barriers, they are not insurmountable.

—-

Case Study: Laura and Tim's Communication Struggles

Laura, a 35-year-old project manager, often found herself interrupting her husband Tim mid-sentence. Tim felt frustrated, believing Laura didn't value his thoughts. At the same time, Laura felt ashamed, knowing her interruptions weren't intentional but struggling to stop them.

With time and effort, Laura and Tim developed strategies to address this challenge. Laura started using mindfulness techniques to pause before speaking, while Tim practiced patience and gently reminded Laura when she interrupted. This mutual effort helped them communicate more effectively and reduced the tension in their conversations.

—-

Tools for Better Communication in ADHD Relationships

1. Active Listening: ADHD brains often jump ahead in conversations, thinking of responses before the other person finishes speaking. Practice summarizing what your partner says before responding.

2. Pause and Reflect: Use a mental or physical pause button (like a deep breath or a count to three) before reacting, especially in emotionally charged moments.

3. Set Communication Boundaries: Agree on times for important discussions when both partners are calm and focused. Avoid tackling big issues during moments of stress or distraction.

4. Use Visual Aids: Write down key points or use tools like shared

calendars and lists to reinforce conversations.

—-

The Power of "I" Statements

When emotions run high, it's easy to blame or criticize. Using "I" statements helps frame concerns without putting your partner on the defensive. For example:

Instead of: "You never listen to me!"

Try: "I feel unheard when I'm interrupted during conversations."

This subtle shift fosters understanding and collaboration rather than conflict.

—-

Navigating Conflict with ADHD

Conflict is inevitable in any relationship, but ADHD can amplify disagreements due to impulsivity, emotional intensity, or miscommunication. To navigate conflict effectively:

1. Take Time-Outs: If emotions escalate, agree to take a break and revisit the discussion when both partners are calm.

2. Avoid "Kitchen-Sinking": ADHD brains may bring up multiple unrelated issues during a conflict. Stay focused on one topic at a time.

3. Use Gentle Reminders: Partners can gently point out when ADHD tendencies, like interrupting or zoning out, arise during disagreements.

—-

Case Study: Maya and Conflict Resolution

Maya, a 29-year-old artist, often spiraled into emotional outbursts during arguments with her girlfriend, Alana. She felt overwhelmed by her emotions and struggled to stay focused on the issue at hand.

Through therapy, Maya learned to use a "time-out" strategy. When tensions rose, she and Alana would pause the conversation for 10 minutes. During this time, Maya practiced deep breathing or wrote down her thoughts. These breaks allowed Maya to return to the discussion feeling grounded and better equipped to communicate effectively.

—-

The Role of Rejection Sensitivity Dysphoria (RSD) in Communication

Rejection sensitivity dysphoria, a common experience for

women with ADHD, can distort how they perceive and respond to feedback. Even mild criticism may feel like a personal attack, leading to defensiveness or withdrawal.

To manage RSD in communication:

Acknowledge Your Feelings: Recognize when you're reacting out of rejection sensitivity rather than the actual situation.

Ask for Clarification: Instead of assuming the worst, ask your partner to clarify their intent. For example, "Did you mean X? I'm feeling unsure."

Practice Self-Compassion: Remind yourself that criticism isn't a reflection of your worth but an opportunity for growth.

—-

Leveraging ADHD Strengths in Communication

Despite its challenges, ADHD also brings unique strengths to communication:

1. Empathy: Many ADHD women are deeply attuned to others' emotions, making them supportive and understanding partners.

2. Passion: ADHD brains are wired for intensity, which can translate into heartfelt, enthusiastic conversations.

3. Creativity: ADHD fosters out-of-the-box thinking, helping women find innovative ways to express their thoughts and feelings.

—-

Building Rituals of Connection

Small, consistent communication habits can strengthen intimacy over time. Consider incorporating rituals like:

Daily Check-Ins: Spend 10 minutes each evening sharing highs and lows from your day.

"Love Notes" System: Leave small, written reminders of appreciation or encouragement for your partner.

Weekly Conversations: Dedicate time to discuss any challenges or needs in your relationship, keeping the dialogue open and constructive.

—-

Case Study: Building Communication Habits

Sophie and Aaron, a married couple in their early 40s, struggled to find time for meaningful conversations amidst busy schedules. Sophie, who has ADHD, often forgot to bring up important topics until they escalated into conflicts.

To address this, they introduced a weekly ritual: Sunday coffee chats. During these chats, they reviewed their week, shared any concerns, and planned the upcoming week together. This structured time helped Sophie feel less scattered and allowed Aaron to feel more included in her thought process.

—-

Practical Takeaways for Better Communication

Be Honest About ADHD: Share how ADHD impacts your communication style and encourage your partner to ask questions.

Seek Feedback: Ask your partner how you can communicate more effectively and share how they can support you in return.

Celebrate Progress: Acknowledge improvements in your communication skills, even if they seem small.

—-

From Struggle to Strength

Communication is the cornerstone of intimacy, and for women with ADHD, it requires patience, practice, and self-awareness. By addressing challenges and celebrating strengths, ADHD women can create deeper, more meaningful connections with their partners.

Chapter 6 will explore the emotional roller coaster of ADHD relationships, offering tools for managing emotional intensity and fostering balance.

6

Navigating the Roller Coaster of Emotional Intensity

Living on the Emotional Edge

Women with ADHD often describe their emotional world as a roller coaster—filled with exhilarating highs, devastating lows, and sudden, unpredictable turns. Emotional intensity is a core feature of ADHD, shaping how women experience love, conflict, and connection.

While this intensity can deepen relationships, it can also create challenges when emotions feel overwhelming or difficult to regulate. This chapter explores how women with ADHD can navigate their emotional highs and lows, fostering balance and resilience in their intimate relationships.

—-

Understanding Emotional Intensity in ADHD

ADHD-related emotional intensity stems from differences in how the brain processes and regulates feelings. Common experiences include:

1. Rejection Sensitivity Dysphoria (RSD): A heightened sensitivity to perceived rejection or criticism, leading to disproportionate emotional reactions.

2. Emotional Flooding: Feeling emotions so deeply that they overwhelm logical thinking.

3. Rapid Shifts in Mood: Moving quickly from joy to frustration or sadness, sometimes without a clear trigger.

These emotional patterns can leave partners confused or hurt, particularly if they misinterpret intense reactions as overreacting or instability.

— -

Case Study: Anna's Emotional Flooding

Anna, a 31-year-old with ADHD, found herself crying uncontrollably when her boyfriend, Tom, canceled a dinner date. While Tom saw it as a minor change, Anna felt devastated, interpreting his actions as a sign that he didn't care about her.

Afterward, Anna recognized that her reaction was tied to RSD.

She began using grounding techniques, like deep breathing and journaling, to process her emotions before responding. She also shared her feelings with Tom, explaining how her ADHD influenced her reactions. With time, they developed strategies to navigate these emotional moments together.

— -

Emotional Dysregulation vs. Emotional Depth

It's important to distinguish between emotional dysregulation and emotional depth:

Emotional Dysregulation: Difficulty controlling the intensity or duration of emotions, often leading to impulsive reactions or prolonged distress.

Emotional Depth: The ability to feel emotions deeply and connect with others on a profound level.

While dysregulation can create challenges, emotional depth is a gift that allows ADHD women to form deeply empathetic and passionate bonds.

— -

Tools for Managing Emotional Intensity

1. Pause and Reflect: When emotions feel overwhelming, pause before reacting. Use techniques like deep breathing, counting to 10, or stepping away from the situation.

2. Name the Emotion: Labeling your feelings (e.g., "I'm feeling rejected" or "I'm frustrated") can help you process them more effectively.

3. Use a Sensory Reset: Ground yourself using sensory tools like holding a weighted object, listening to calming music, or taking a warm shower.

4. Practice Emotional Check-Ins: Set aside time each day to reflect on your emotions and identify patterns or triggers.

— -

Navigating Emotional Dysregulation in Relationships

Emotional dysregulation can create tension in intimate relationships, particularly when partners don't understand its roots. To navigate these challenges:

Communicate During Calm Moments: Share how ADHD influences your emotions when both you and your partner are calm.

Establish Conflict Protocols: Agree on strategies for handling emotional moments, such as taking time-outs or using code words to de-escalate tension.

Focus on Repair: After an emotional outburst, prioritize repairing the connection through apology, reassurance, and understanding.

—-

Case Study: Emily's Conflict Protocol

Emily, a 40-year-old teacher with ADHD, often found herself yelling during arguments with her wife, Rachel. These outbursts left Rachel feeling hurt and disconnected.

Together, they developed a conflict protocol: When tensions rose, Emily would step outside for five minutes to calm down. Rachel, meanwhile, would write down her thoughts to organize her response. These small changes helped them approach conflicts with greater clarity and compassion.

—-

Grounding Techniques for Emotional Regulation

Grounding techniques are tools that help women with ADHD reconnect with the present moment during emotional dysregulation. Some effective strategies include:

1. The 5-4-3-2-1 Method: Identify five things you can see, four things you can touch, three things you can hear, two things you can smell, and one thing you can taste.

2. Breathing Exercises: Practice deep breathing, such as inhaling for four counts, holding for four counts, and exhaling for four counts.

3. Progressive Muscle Relaxation: Tense and release each muscle group in your body, starting with your toes and moving upward.

—-

Rejection Sensitivity Dysphoria (RSD) and Its Impact

RSD can make women with ADHD hypersensitive to perceived rejection, even when none exists. This sensitivity often leads to:

Overanalyzing Partner Behavior: Reading into small actions, like a delayed text reply, as signs of disinterest.

Avoidance: Withdrawing from intimacy to avoid potential rejection.

Intense Reactions: Responding with anger, tears, or shutdowns when feeling rejected.

To manage RSD in relationships:

Challenge Negative Thoughts: Ask yourself, "What evidence do I have that my partner is rejecting me?"

Communicate Needs Clearly: Let your partner know how RSD affects you and what reassurance you might need.

Seek Validation from Yourself: Practice self-affirmations to counter feelings of rejection.

—-

Case Study: Managing RSD with Support

Sophia, a 28-year-old software engineer with ADHD, often felt anxious when her partner, Alex, seemed distracted during their conversations. She interpreted his behavior as disinterest, triggering feelings of rejection.

With Alex's support, Sophia started challenging her negative thoughts by journaling evidence of their strong relationship. Alex, in turn, made an effort to validate Sophia's feelings by giving her his full attention during conversations.

—-

Fostering Emotional Balance in Relationships

While emotional intensity is a natural part of ADHD, balance can be cultivated through:

1. Self-Awareness: Regularly reflect on your emotions and identify patterns in your reactions.

2. Healthy Outlets: Channel intense emotions into creative pursuits, physical activity, or mindfulness practices.

3. Support Systems: Lean on trusted friends, therapists, or support groups for validation and perspective.

—-

Celebrating Emotional Strengths

Women with ADHD often bring unique emotional strengths to their relationships, including:

Passion: The ability to love deeply and express affection wholeheartedly.

Empathy: A profound capacity to understand and share a partner's feelings.

Resilience: The ability to grow and adapt, even in the face of emotional challenges.

By embracing these strengths, ADHD women can transform their emotional intensity into a source of connection and growth.

—-

Riding the Roller Coaster Together

Emotional intensity is both a challenge and a gift for women with ADHD. By learning to manage their emotional highs and lows, they can foster intimacy that is both passionate and balanced.

Chapter 7 will explore how hormones influence ADHD and intimacy, offering insights into how women can navigate these changes with self-compassion and understanding.

7

The Hormonal Puzzle

For women with ADHD, hormones can feel like an unpredictable force that amplifies emotions, energy levels, and even sensory sensitivity. Hormonal fluctuations throughout the menstrual cycle, pregnancy, postpartum, and menopause have profound effects on ADHD symptoms and, by extension, intimacy.

Understanding how hormones interact with ADHD is critical for managing relationships and fostering connection. In this chapter, we'll explore the hormonal journey and offer strategies for navigating these changes with self-compassion and clarity.

—-

The Hormonal Connection to ADHD

ADHD symptoms are deeply influenced by hormones, particularly estrogen. Estrogen plays a key role in regulating dopamine, the neurotransmitter associated with attention and reward. As estrogen levels fluctuate, so do ADHD symptoms.

High Estrogen Levels: During ovulation, higher estrogen levels may temporarily improve focus, mood, and energy.

Low Estrogen Levels: Before menstruation or during menopause, lower estrogen levels can worsen ADHD symptoms, leading to irritability, distractibility, and emotional dysregulation.

These hormonal shifts can also affect intimacy by altering mood, libido, and the ability to connect emotionally or physically.

— -

The Menstrual Cycle and ADHD

The menstrual cycle creates a predictable pattern of hormonal changes that impact ADHD symptoms and intimacy.

1. Follicular Phase (Day 1–14): Estrogen levels gradually rise, improving focus and energy. Women may feel more confident and emotionally available.

2. Ovulation (Around Day 14): Peak estrogen levels often lead to heightened libido and a desire for connection.

3. Luteal Phase (Day 15–28): Estrogen drops while progesterone rises. ADHD symptoms like forgetfulness, irritability, and emotional intensity may increase.

4. Menstrual Phase (Days 1–5 of the next cycle): Hormone levels reset, often accompanied by fatigue and sensory sensitivity.

For women with ADHD, the luteal phase can be particularly challenging, as low estrogen amplifies symptoms like emotional dysregulation and rejection sensitivity.

—-

Case Study: Lily's Monthly Roller Coaster

Lily, a 30-year-old with ADHD, noticed a pattern in her relationship with her partner, Sam. During the week before her period, she became unusually irritable and distant, often misinterpreting Sam's actions as rejection.

After tracking her menstrual cycle, Lily identified this pattern as part of her luteal phase. She shared her findings with Sam, who began offering extra patience and reassurance during these times. Lily also scheduled self-care activities during her luteal phase, like yoga and journaling, to help manage her emotions.

—-

Pregnancy and Postpartum ADHD

Pregnancy introduces dramatic hormonal shifts that can impact ADHD symptoms and intimacy.

Pregnancy: Some women experience a temporary reduction in ADHD symptoms due to higher estrogen levels, while others find pregnancy exacerbates their struggles with focus and emotional regulation.

Postpartum: After childbirth, estrogen levels plummet, often intensifying ADHD symptoms. Sleep deprivation and the demands of a newborn can add to this challenge, creating strain on intimate relationships.

Strategies for Pregnancy and Postpartum:

Communicate Needs: Share your emotional and physical challenges with your partner to foster understanding.

Simplify Tasks: Reduce household or social obligations to focus on recovery and connection.

Seek Professional Support: Work with a therapist or healthcare provider to address postpartum ADHD challenges.

—-

Case Study: Navigating Postpartum with ADHD

Sara, a 35-year-old mother with ADHD, felt overwhelmed after the birth of her daughter. She became forgetful, irritable, and disconnected from her husband, Mark, who misinterpreted her behavior as a lack of interest in their relationship.

With the help of a therapist, Sara and Mark created a plan to share responsibilities and prioritize their connection. They introduced a nightly ritual of sharing gratitude, even if it was just one sentence each, to maintain emotional closeness during this demanding time.

—-

ADHD and Menopause

Menopause brings a significant decline in estrogen levels, which can worsen ADHD symptoms. Women may notice increased forgetfulness, emotional dysregulation, and difficulty focusing. These changes can affect intimacy by reducing energy levels and libido.

Tips for Navigating Menopause:

Track Symptoms: Use a journal to identify patterns in mood, energy, and focus.

Consider Hormonal Therapy: Discuss options like hormone replacement therapy (HRT) with a healthcare provider.

Prioritize Restorative Activities: Engage in activities that replenish energy and reduce stress, like mindfulness, exercise, or creative hobbies.

—-

Case Study: Rekindling Intimacy During Menopause

Amara, a 50-year-old with ADHD, noticed a decline in her

libido and energy during menopause, which created distance in her marriage to Daniel. She felt embarrassed discussing her struggles, fearing Daniel would lose interest.

After opening up, Amara and Daniel explored new ways to connect, such as taking dance classes and scheduling intimate moments during her high-energy periods. Amara also began hormone replacement therapy, which improved her mood and focus.

—-

Managing Hormonal Shifts in Relationships

To navigate the impact of hormones on ADHD and intimacy:

1. Educate Your Partner: Share how hormonal changes affect your mood, energy, and ADHD symptoms.

2. Track Patterns: Use apps or journals to monitor your cycle and predict challenging phases.

3. Plan for Self-Care: Schedule rest, relaxation, and enjoyable activities during low-energy or high-sensitivity periods.

4. Communicate Early and Often: Discuss hormonal shifts proactively to prevent misunderstandings or conflicts.

—-

Celebrating the Strengths of Change

While hormonal changes can create challenges, they also offer opportunities for growth and connection:

Self-Awareness: Understanding how hormones affect ADHD empowers women to make informed decisions about their needs.

Adaptability: Navigating these changes together strengthens resilience and intimacy in relationships.

Deeper Connection: Sharing vulnerabilities fosters emotional closeness and mutual support.

—-

Embracing the Hormonal Journey

Hormones are an integral part of the ADHD experience for women, shaping both their personal and relational lives. By understanding and working with these shifts, women can navigate intimacy with greater compassion and confidence.

Chapter 8 will explore how parenthood impacts ADHD and relationships, offering insights into balancing caregiving, self-care, and intimacy.

8

Parenthood, ADHD, and Relationship Dynamics

The Triple Load

Parenthood is a transformative experience, bringing immense joy and challenges. For women with ADHD, the demands of parenting, managing their ADHD symptoms, and maintaining a healthy relationship can feel overwhelming. Balancing these responsibilities often requires creativity, self-awareness, and teamwork.

In this chapter, we'll explore the unique challenges ADHD moms face in parenting and relationships, while offering strategies to nurture intimacy and shared responsibilities amidst the chaos of family life.

—-

The Impact of Parenthood on ADHD and Relationships

Parenthood introduces new complexities to ADHD and intimacy:

1. Increased Mental Load: The executive function challenges of ADHD make managing schedules, schoolwork, and household tasks more taxing.

2. Time and Energy Constraints: Parenting leaves little time for self-care or nurturing romantic relationships.

3. Heightened Emotions: ADHD's emotional intensity can amplify feelings of guilt, frustration, or inadequacy as a parent or partner.

4. Shifted Priorities: Couples may focus solely on parenting, neglecting their own relationship.

While these challenges can strain relationships, they also create opportunities for growth and deeper connection when addressed collaboratively.

—-

Case Study: Priya and Balancing Parenting with ADHD

Priya, a 36-year-old mother of two, struggled to keep up with her family's busy schedule. Her ADHD made it hard to remember appointments and keep the house organized, which led to frequent arguments with her husband, Arun.

Feeling overwhelmed, Priya enlisted Arun's help to divide responsibilities more equitably. They created a shared digital calendar and a weekly family meeting to review tasks. Arun also began encouraging Priya to take breaks for self-care, which improved her energy and focus. These changes strengthened their partnership and reduced tension in their marriage.

—-

ADHD Strengths in Parenting

While ADHD presents challenges, it also equips women with unique strengths as parents:

1. Creativity: ADHD moms excel at finding fun, innovative ways to engage their children.

2. Empathy: Emotional depth helps them connect with their kids on a meaningful level.

3. Spontaneity: An adventurous spirit brings joy and excitement to family life.

4. Adaptability: ADHD moms are skilled at thinking on their feet

and adjusting to changing circumstances.

Recognizing and leveraging these strengths can help ADHD moms feel more confident in their parenting abilities.

— -

Strategies for Balancing ADHD, Parenting, and Intimacy

1. Share the Load: Divide parenting and household responsibilities equitably with your partner. Use tools like shared calendars, chore charts, or task management apps to stay organized.

2. Set Realistic Expectations: Accept that perfection isn't the goal. Focus on what truly matters, and let go of guilt about less-important tasks.

3. Carve Out Couple Time: Prioritize moments for connection, even if it's just a quick check-in or a shared cup of coffee after the kids are in bed.

4. Involve Your Partner: Communicate openly about your ADHD challenges and how your partner can support you.

— -

Case Study: Sophie's "Parenting Team" Approach

Sophie, a 38-year-old with ADHD, often felt like she was failing as a mom and partner. She struggled to keep her three kids' schedules straight and felt disconnected from her husband, Matt.

After a particularly tough week, Sophie and Matt sat down to reassess their approach. They created a "parenting team" system, dividing tasks based on their strengths—Sophie handled creative projects and emotional support, while Matt managed logistics like scheduling and bills. This division of labor lightened Sophie's mental load and allowed the couple to spend more quality time together.

The Role of Self-Care in Balancing ADHD and Parenthood

Self-care is essential for managing ADHD and maintaining intimacy. ADHD moms often put their family's needs first, but neglecting their own well-being can lead to burnout.

Simple Self-Care Ideas:

Mindfulness Moments: Take five minutes daily to practice deep breathing or meditation.

Movement Breaks: Engage in physical activity, like yoga or a brisk walk, to recharge.

Creative Outlets: Use hobbies or journaling to process emotions and reduce stress.

Ask for Help: Delegate tasks or lean on your support network when needed.

— -

Navigating Emotional Dysregulation as a Parent

Parenting often tests emotional regulation, especially for women with ADHD. To navigate emotional moments:

1. Pause and Reflect: If you feel overwhelmed, step away from the situation to collect your thoughts.

2. Model Emotional Regulation: Share your strategies with your kids, like saying, "I'm feeling frustrated, so I'm going to take a deep breath before we talk."

3. Repair After Outbursts: If you lose your temper, apologize and explain your feelings. This teaches kids the importance of accountability and communication.

— -

Balancing Co-Parenting Dynamics

Co-parenting with ADHD adds another layer of complexity, as partners may have different parenting styles or expectations. To balance these dynamics:

Communicate Regularly: Hold weekly check-ins to discuss parenting strategies, challenges, and successes.

Focus on Strengths: Divide responsibilities based on each partner's strengths and preferences.

Celebrate Wins Together: Acknowledge your teamwork and the positive impact on your family.

—-

Case Study: Emma and James' Co-Parenting Success

Emma, a 42-year-old with ADHD, often clashed with her husband, James, over their parenting styles. Emma thrived on spontaneity, while James preferred structure. Their differences created tension, especially during stressful times.

After discussing their frustrations, Emma and James decided to align their parenting goals. They agreed on a mix of structure and flexibility, setting routines for essential tasks while leaving room for fun and creativity. This compromise improved their teamwork and brought more harmony to their home.

—-

Rekindling Intimacy After Parenthood

Parenthood can shift focus away from romantic relationships, but rekindling intimacy is possible with intentional effort:

1. Schedule Date Nights: Even if it's just watching a movie at home, prioritize time for connection.

2. Express Gratitude: Regularly acknowledge your partner's efforts, whether it's for parenting or supporting your ADHD journey.

3. Rediscover Each Other: Share your thoughts, dreams, and interests outside of parenting roles to nurture your bond.

—-

Celebrating the Joys of Parenting with ADHD

Parenting with ADHD is a journey of ups and downs, but it's also filled with unique joys:

Shared Adventures: Spontaneous outings or creative projects create lasting memories.

Empathy and Understanding: ADHD moms often raise children who feel deeply seen and loved.

Resilience as a Team: Navigating challenges together strengthens the family bond.

Conclusion: Embracing the Parenting Journey

Parenthood with ADHD requires flexibility, communication, and self-compassion. By leveraging strengths, sharing responsibilities, and prioritizing intimacy, ADHD moms can balance their roles as caregivers, partners, and individuals.

Chapter 9 will focus on leveraging ADHD strengths for deeper connections, celebrating the unique qualities that women with ADHD bring to their relationships.

9

Leveraging ADHD Strengths for Deeper Connections

The Power of Perspective

Women with ADHD often focus on the challenges their condition brings to relationships—forgetfulness, impulsivity, or emotional intensity. But ADHD also gifts women with unique strengths that can enhance intimacy and connection. Creativity, empathy, and a zest for life are just a few of the qualities that make ADHD women extraordinary partners.

This chapter explores how to shift the narrative from struggle to strength, highlighting the ways ADHD can enrich relationships and create deeper bonds.

—-

The Strengths of ADHD in Relationships

LEVERAGING ADHD STRENGTHS FOR DEEPER CONNECTIONS

ADHD women bring unique qualities to their relationships that foster connection and joy:

1. Creativity: ADHD brains excel at thinking outside the box, turning ordinary moments into memorable experiences.

2. Empathy: Deep emotional sensitivity allows ADHD women to tune into their partner's feelings, fostering understanding and compassion.

3. Passion: ADHD's intensity often translates into enthusiasm and dedication, fueling vibrant, exciting relationships.

4. Spontaneity: An adventurous spirit keeps relationships dynamic and fun, creating a sense of excitement and unpredictability.

5. Resilience: ADHD women are masters of adaptation, navigating challenges with determination and creativity.

—-

Case Study: Mia's Creative Spark

Mia, a 29-year-old artist with ADHD, often felt insecure about her distractibility and disorganization in her relationship with her boyfriend, Sam. She worried these traits overshadowed her ability to be a good partner.

One day, Sam mentioned feeling stressed about work. Inspired by her creativity, Mia planned a surprise picnic in their living room, complete with fairy lights and homemade snacks. Sam was moved by Mia's thoughtfulness, and the experience reminded Mia of the unique joy she brings to their relationship.

—-

Harnessing ADHD Strengths for Connection

1. Lean Into Creativity: Use your ADHD-driven creativity to plan meaningful activities or surprise your partner with thoughtful gestures. Examples include:

Crafting a personalized gift, like a scrapbook or playlist.

Planning a spontaneous day trip or date night.

2. Celebrate Empathy: Channel your emotional depth into meaningful conversations. For instance:

Practice active listening, reflecting your partner's feelings to show understanding.

Use your empathy to support your partner during tough times, offering reassurance and encouragement.

3. Embrace Spontaneity: Let your natural enthusiasm create moments of joy and adventure in your relationship. Examples include:

Suggesting an impromptu outing, like stargazing or dancing in the kitchen.

Turning mundane activities into games or shared experiences.

Case Study: Elena's Spontaneous Adventures

Elena, a 34-year-old with ADHD, loved surprising her wife, Rachel, with impromptu plans. One weekend, Elena suggested they pack a bag and take a road trip to a nearby beach town. Though Rachel initially hesitated, the trip turned out to be one of their most cherished memories, full of laughter and connection.

By embracing her spontaneous nature, Elena added excitement and vibrancy to their relationship.

Balancing Strengths with Challenges

While ADHD strengths bring vibrancy to relationships, they must be balanced with intentionality to avoid overwhelming your partner.

1. Channel Energy Purposefully: Use your enthusiasm to support your partner's goals, like cheering them on during a big project or helping them relax after a stressful day.

2. Set Boundaries for Spontaneity: Ensure your spontaneous plans align with your partner's energy levels and commitments.

3. Build Systems for Follow-Through: Use reminders or shared calendars to ensure your creative ideas come to fruition, demonstrating reliability alongside creativity.

—-

Reframing ADHD in Your Relationship

Shifting the narrative around ADHD from "burden" to "strength" can transform how you and your partner view your dynamic. Strategies for reframing include:

Focus on Positives: Highlight the ways your ADHD traits—like passion or empathy—enhance your connection.

Acknowledge Growth: Celebrate moments when you've used ADHD strengths to navigate challenges.

Involve Your Partner: Invite your partner to share how your unique traits positively impact your relationship.

Case Study: Rewriting the ADHD Narrative

Sofia, a 31-year-old teacher with ADHD, often apologized to her husband, Mark, for her forgetfulness or emotional outbursts. Over time, Mark helped Sofia reframe these moments, reminding her of the countless times her creativity and enthusiasm had brought joy to their family.

Together, they began focusing on the strengths ADHD brought to their relationship, creating a new, empowering narrative that deepened their bond.

Strength-Based Communication

Highlighting strengths in communication fosters positivity and collaboration. Examples include:

1. Acknowledging Effort: Instead of focusing on challenges, celebrate progress. For example, "I love how you made dinner tonight—it felt so thoughtful."

2. Sharing Gratitude: Regularly express appreciation for your partner's support and the ways they contribute to your relationship.

3. Building on Strengths: Encourage each other to use your unique abilities, like creativity or problem-solving, to navigate challenges.

—-

Case Study: Celebrating Strengths

Nina, a 38-year-old with ADHD, often felt guilty about needing reminders for household tasks. Her partner, Alex, reframed this by acknowledging Nina's strengths: "You're incredible at planning our family celebrations. I'm happy to remind you about the laundry if it means we get those magical moments you create."

This shift in perspective allowed Nina to focus on her strengths rather than dwelling on her struggles.

—-

Creating a Strength-Focused Relationship

To cultivate a relationship that celebrates ADHD strengths:

1. Reflect on Shared Wins: Regularly discuss moments where ADHD traits—like creativity or resilience—brought joy or solved a problem.

2. Integrate Strengths into Rituals: Use your creativity and empathy to design rituals, like weekly check-ins or shared

hobbies, that strengthen your bond.

3. Celebrate Uniqueness: Embrace the quirks and qualities that make your relationship distinct.

— -

Thriving Together

ADHD brings unique challenges, but it also gifts women with extraordinary strengths that can deepen intimacy and connection. By celebrating these strengths and balancing them with intentional effort, women with ADHD can create relationships that thrive on authenticity, creativity, and love.

Chapter 10 will explore how to heal, grow, and thrive together, offering tools for building a sustainable, fulfilling partnership.

10

Healing, Growth, and Thriving Together

The Journey Forward

Navigating intimacy and relationships as a woman with ADHD is a journey of learning, unlearning, and growth. Challenges like emotional dysregulation, impulsivity, or forgetfulness can strain relationships, but they also offer opportunities for healing and resilience.

This chapter focuses on the final leg of this journey: embracing imperfection, fostering growth, and creating a partnership built on mutual understanding and love. Thriving together isn't about eliminating challenges—it's about transforming them into opportunities for connection.

—-

Healing as an ADHD Woman

Healing begins with self-compassion. Many women with

ADHD carry years of guilt or shame, often rooted in societal expectations or past relationships. Recognizing that ADHD is a part of your identity—not a flaw—can be transformative.

Steps Toward Healing:

1. Acknowledge Your Journey: Reflect on the unique challenges you've faced and the strengths you've developed along the way.

2. Challenge Negative Self-Talk: Replace self-criticism with affirmations that celebrate your progress and resilience.

3. Seek Professional Support: Therapy or coaching can help you process past experiences and develop tools for thriving in relationships.

— -

Case Study: Rekindling Self-Compassion

After years of feeling like a "bad partner" because of her forgetfulness, Jasmine, a 32-year-old with ADHD, began working with a therapist. Through therapy, she realized that her partner valued her creativity and enthusiasm far more than the occasional forgotten date.

Jasmine started journaling her strengths and revisiting this list whenever self-doubt crept in. This practice helped her approach her relationship with greater confidence and authenticity.

Growing Together: Building Resilience as a Couple

Growth in relationships happens when both partners are committed to understanding and supporting each other. For women with ADHD, this means fostering an environment of empathy, collaboration, and shared goals.

Strategies for Growing Together:

1. Celebrate Small Wins: Acknowledge everyday successes, like working through a conflict or completing a shared task, to build momentum.

2. Set Relationship Goals: Work together to identify areas for growth, such as improving communication or planning more quality time.

3. Learn Each Other's Triggers: Understanding what triggers emotional reactions in both partners helps prevent conflicts and foster patience.

Case Study: Emily and Zach's Growth Plan

Emily, a 35-year-old with ADHD, often felt overwhelmed by her partner Zach's need for structure. Zach, in turn, struggled to adjust to Emily's spontaneous nature. They decided to create a "growth plan" for their relationship, focusing on:

Scheduling one structured date night (Zach's preference) and one spontaneous outing (Emily's preference) each month.

Practicing active listening during disagreements.

Celebrating their strengths by acknowledging how Zach's organization complemented Emily's creativity.

This intentional approach helped Emily and Zach grow closer while honoring their differences.

— -

Thriving Together: Sustaining Connection Over Time

Thriving in a relationship requires consistent effort and adaptability. Life's challenges—parenthood, career changes, or aging—will inevitably test your partnership. By grounding your relationship in shared values and mutual support, you can weather these changes together.

Keys to Thriving Together:

1. Prioritize Connection: Regularly invest time in nurturing your bond, whether through date nights, shared hobbies, or meaningful conversations.

2. Adapt to Change: Recognize that ADHD traits—and your relationship—will evolve over time. Stay flexible and open to new strategies for connection.

3. Practice Gratitude: Express appreciation for your partner's efforts, celebrating the ways they support and love you.

The Role of Forgiveness in Thriving Relationships

Forgiveness is a cornerstone of thriving relationships, particularly when ADHD-related challenges create friction. This includes forgiving yourself for mistakes, as well as fostering a culture of forgiveness within your relationship.

How to Practice Forgiveness:

Acknowledge Harm: Recognize when actions or behaviors have caused pain, and address them openly.

Take Accountability: Apologize sincerely, and outline steps to prevent repeating the mistake.

Let Go of Resentment: Focus on growth and progress rather than dwelling on past mistakes.

Case Study: Forgiving and Moving Forward

Maya, a 40-year-old with ADHD, forgot her anniversary with her husband, Alex, two years in a row. Alex felt hurt, interpreting Maya's forgetfulness as a lack of care.

After a heartfelt conversation, Maya apologized and explained how her ADHD contributed to the oversight. She created a system of reminders to ensure she didn't forget important dates in the future. Alex, seeing Maya's effort, chose to forgive her and focus on the many ways she showed love in their everyday life.

—-

Celebrating Your Unique Partnership

Every relationship involving ADHD is unique, shaped by the strengths and challenges both partners bring to the table. By celebrating what makes your partnership special, you can foster a sense of pride and joy in your connection.

Ways to Celebrate Your Partnership:

Create Shared Rituals: Develop traditions that reflect your bond, like an annual getaway or a monthly gratitude practice.

Honor Milestones: Celebrate not just anniversaries, but also achievements like resolving a conflict or supporting each other through a tough time.

Share Your Story: Reflect on how your journey together has shaped you, strengthening your bond and inspiring others.

Case Study: Strengthening a Unique Bond

Sofia and Liam, a couple navigating ADHD, made a tradition of writing each other letters on their anniversary. These letters highlighted their favorite memories from the past year and the ways they'd supported each other through challenges.

This simple practice reminded them of their growth as a couple and helped them stay connected, even during difficult times.

Thriving in Love and Life

Thriving in a relationship as a woman with ADHD isn't about perfection—it's about embracing the journey, celebrating your strengths, and committing to growth. By fostering self-compassion, building resilience together, and nurturing your unique connection, you can create a partnership that thrives on love, understanding, and joy.

This is just the beginning of your journey toward deeper intimacy and connection. Continue to explore, adapt, and celebrate the extraordinary bond you share with your partner.

Final Note to the Reader

Thank you for joining this exploration of ADHD and intimacy.

Your experiences and strengths are a testament to the beauty of connection in all its forms. May this book inspire you to embrace your ADHD as a source of resilience and love, creating relationships that are as unique and extraordinary as you are.

www.ingramcontent.com/pod-product-compliance
Lightning Source LLC
Chambersburg PA
CBHW071725020426
42333CB00017B/2397